SUGAR for DIABETICS

Cure DIABETES type 2 with STEVIA

Reduce blood sugar naturally

Dr. Matt Roberts

Published by:

JoelNoah S.A.

info@joelnoah.com

Author: Dr. Matt Roberts

Sugar for diabetics - Cure diabetes type 2 with stevia

Reduce blood sugar naturally

ISBN-13: 978-1493738021

ISBN-10: 149373802X

Copyright 2013 by JoelNoah S.A.

INDEX

Introduction

Diabetes is a disease of our civilization. Worldwide approximately 350 million people are affected; this number continues increasing every year.

In this context, during the last few years there has been more and more talk of a plant which has extraordinary properties for diabetes disease. It has an extreme natural sweetening, without harmful side effects. With it, it is possible to marvelously improve the condition of people with diabetes type 2, and to achieve real miracles when it comes to losing weight.

The plant, originally from South America, has the botanic name Stevia rebaudiana Bertoni; its common name is stevia, and it belongs to the family of Composites (Asteraceae). It is also known as sweet weed, sweet leaf, sugar hat or honey weed. Today, 150-300 species are known. It is originally from the Amambay Mountains, in the border region between Paraguay and Brazil.

It is known to the indigenous people of South America for many centuries, due to its sweetening effect and its medical properties. Several tribes of Indians use stevia to sweeten their *mate* tea and their foods. As a medicine, they use it to cure wounds and for diabetes.

The Guaraní people in Paraguay and Brazil are not familiar with overweight, diabetes, or skin problems.

The plant was mentioned as early as the 16th Century from Spanish conquerors, and investigated in 1887 from Moises Giacomo Bertoni from Switzerland. He gave the plant its current name, in 1905.

Classification of the diabetes types

Diabetes mellitus (Greek for honey-sweet flow) is basically subdivided into types 1, 2, 3, and 4.

Diabetes mellitus type 1

Type 1 was formerly called juvenile diabetes (meaning youth diabetes). It is further subdivided into types 1a and 1b. 1a is the type obtained through immunity, for example LADA (a special type of diabetes mellitus type 1 – LADA), while type 1b represents the idiopathic form, i.e., there is no discernible cause.

In 70-80% of the cases, the disease appears before the age of 35. Basically the disease can appear at any age.

This is an auto-immune disease, in which the so-called B-cells of the pancreas are progressively destroyed. Antibodies against B-cells can be found. The B-cells of the pancreas produce insulin. Insulin is a special protein which acts as a hormone. Its task is to reduce the increased blood sugar level after ingesting food. This happens because insulin carries out a key role: the sugar in the blood is taken into the body cells by the insulin, especially muscle and liver cells. There, the sugar is initially stored, and if required, activated again, making it available as an energy carrier. Thus, it is clear that when the B-cells are destroyed, no more insulin can be produced and the blood's sugar content increases.

For this disease, a genetic predisposition was detected (a genetic predisposition refers to a hereditary trait, or a high probability to get certain diseases). However, less than 10% of other family members get diabetes type 1. Apart from the genetic predisposition, there must be additional factors, for example a rubella infection. Such an infection may have occurred several years in the past.

Patients normally have a regular weight. The disease starts acutely and can be provoked by a current metabolic stress, for example an infection or operation. Patients lose weight dramatically even when eating normally, they feel languid, complain of tiredness, have a lot of thirst and also urinate a lot. There can be a diabetic coma. Later in the diseases there is a complete destruction of the B-cells, and the insulin production stops completely. These patients depend on insulin therapy for the rest of their lives.

Subtype diabetes mellitus type 1 – LADA

A type 1 diabetes which appears after an age of 30 is called "latent autoimmune diabetes mellitus in adults" (LADA).

The progress of the disease is slower. There are the typical symptoms of excess sugar. Initially, the insulin production is still sufficient, and the insulin deficiency can be compensated with tablets (typically sulfonylureas). Once the disease continues progressing, the patients require insulin.

In the case of LADA, antibodies against B-cells can also be detected. The probability of getting additional autoimmune diseases (for example, of the thyroid gland) is high.

Diabetes mellitus type 2

In type 2, there are different combinations of insulin resistance, "hyperinsulinism", a relative lack of insulin and secretion failures. This type is further subdivided into type 2a without overweight (obesity) and type 2b with overweight.

Ca. 90% of all diabetics suffer from type 2. This is a genetic disease in which several gene locations are affected. There must also be additional factors, such as overweight. Thus, being overweight is considered to be an increased risk to get diabetes. Frequently, in families with diabetes type 2, several family members have it. When both parents have diabetes, their children have a 70-80% chance of getting diabetes as well.

For the disease to appear, two factors are important:

First: There is an insulin resistance. That means that the effect of insulin is affected. Sugar = glucose is not stored in its pure form, but as glucagon. If glucose is now required as an energy carrier, the liver's energy reserve can convert the glucagon into glucose. This process is called gluconeogenesis.

In the case of insulin resistance, there is an increase in gluconeogenesis, while less glucose gets to the body's cells, remaining instead in the blood. The result is an increased blood sugar content.

Second: The insulin secretion is affected (a relative lack of insulin). Compared to the blood sugar content, too little insulin is released. However, in absolute terms the insulin production is very high.

Both factors affect one another in a vicious circle: if there is insulin resistance, an increased amount of insulin is secreted. The large amount of insulin, in turn, increases the insulin resistance. Type 2 diabetics suffer both problems, so it isn't clear which of the problems is decisive for the disease.

Diabetes type 3

Diabetes type 3 is subdivided into 8 subtypes. Thus, type 3a is caused by genetic defects of the B-cells in the pancreas. Type 3b presents genetic defects in the insulin release. Type 3c presents a diseased or destroyed pancreas. Type 3d is caused by hormonal problems, and type 3e is caused by medication (for example by immune suppressants or glucocorticoids). Type 3f is caused by infectious diseases, type 3g by immune disorders (rare forms), and finally type 3h by other genetic diseases, for example Down syndrome, Huntington's disease and others, which often have diabetes.

Diabetes type 4

Diabetes type 4 is the gestation diabetes. This form of diabetes appears for the first time during pregnancy as diabetes type 1 or type 2, but more frequently as a glucose tolerance disorder. Typically, after giving birth the sugar balance is normalized once again. There are known risk factors that may cause gestation diabetes, but these must not necessarily be present. The risk factors include a genetic predisposition toward diabetes mellitus, an age above 30 years and overweight.

Diabetes and overweight

Overweight is not only a risk factor to get diabetes in the first place; due to the overweight there is the additional risk of having a fat balance disorder. Other problems caused by late diabetes can also be attributed to the overweight.

The late effects of diabetes are fatal. They include heart attacks (the most frequent cause of death), strokes, getting blind (retinopathy), kidney disease as well as leg and foot amputations. Approximately one-third of all dialysis patients are diabetics.

Losing weight will help in any case to require less insulin. In the case of type 2 diabetics, an insulin therapy with medication may even get superfluous. Regular medical checks and an appropriate nutrition are still required, since the diabetes disease is not cured.

Metabolic imbalances should be recognized and treated early.

What special ingredients does the stevia plant have?

It is mainly the plant's leaves that are used. The leaves are processed fresh or dried, or extracts are obtained. Over 100 ingredients are already known; the sweetening ingredients are economically significant.

The sweetening capacity of the stevia plant is enormous. Depending on the climate conditions in which it grows, in the unprocessed form it has 10-30 times the sweetness of our refined sugar; concentrated, it gets up to 300-400 times as sweet. Due to its healthy ingredients, it is an alternative to the unhealthy refined sugar and to chemical sweeteners, some of which are quite harmful.

Stevia has no calories. This makes stevia a good alternative for people who watch out for calories, and especially for diabetics.

The sweetening power comes from the complex molecule stevioside, a glucoside. The glucoside consists of glucose, steviol and sophorose. In 1931, 8 glycosides could be found, which cause the sweet taste. Additional important glycosides apart from stevioside include rebaudioside A, rebaudioside C, and dulcoside A. In the dry mass of a leaf from a plant in the wild, stevioside makes up between 4.5% and 8.4%.

Additional ingredients include especially terpenes and flavonoids. These ingredients are known for their cancer retardant properties.

Another ingredient is a small amount of B-sitosterole. This ingredient has been used for several decades in the therapy for hypercholesterolemia.

Hypercholesterolemia refers to a high cholesterol level in the blood.

Stevia is especially valuable since the plant contains almost all B-vitamins, vitamin C, trace elements, alkaloids and diterpenes.

The callus contains small amount of rutin. Rutin has positive properties for the health of blood vessels, especially the veins.

The benefits of stevia for people with diabetes

Sugar is strictly speaking a poison, therefore it is being considered to introduce measures against a high consumption level, for example making sweets much more expensive.

Stevia is not only harmless, but in the future it can have a significant contribution to avoiding or alleviating diabetes. The stevia plant has the following general benefits:

Stevia has no calories.

It is a natural substance.

Stevia is completely harmless for one's health.

Stevia improves the taste, and doesn't cause dependency on sweet things.

Stevia is appropriate for baking, since the substance can withstand heat up to 200 °C.

Stevia need not be fermented.

Due to the high level of sweetness, a small amount is sufficient.

Stevia assists the digestion.

Stevia is the optimal food supplement for diabetics.

Stevia reduces the appetite for sweet things and fatty foods, as well as the desire to consume alcohol and tobacco.

The first studies about the plant were published by Bertoni in 1899. Since then, research has been done all over the world, especially in Japan, Australia, New Zealand, but also in Europe (Switzerland). In the end, these studies have caused the plant to be allowed in the European Union.

Up to what dose is stevia beneficial for health?

"All things are poison, and nothing is without poison; only the dose makes that a thing not be a poison" – this quote by Paracelsus (Swiss physician, alchemist, mystic and philosopher, 1493-1541) is applicable to all foods and environmental influences (such as sunbathing) or activities (such as sports). Even water as a drink, a necessary solvent, is damaging if 10 liters of it are drunk quickly (this causes hyponatremia).

In 1992, there was a study which determined a daily dose of 7.9 mg of stevioside per kilogram of body weight. For a person with a weight of 70 kg, this would mean that the limit of daily intake would be 553 mg. If you assume that the complete sugar requirements for one day would be replaced by stevioside, this would result in an amount of 130 grams sugar, which would be replaced by 433 mg of stevioside. This assumes a sweetening factor of 300.

A complete substitution is not possible (fructose in fruits and vegetables, lactose in milk / dairy products or the conversion by the body from carbohydrates/fats into sugar cannot be replaced). Thus, you will never consume 433 mg of stevioside.

Other studies determined that even an intake of 20 mg per kg of body weight was harmless, and calculated with a safety factor of 100.

Japanese and Brazilian studies concluded that a daily intake of less than 38.5 mg/kg body weight is harmless; in any case they didn't determine a toxic effect.

The European offices of food safety are especially careful; in April 2010 they declared a daily amount of 4 mg stevioside per kilogram of body weight to be harmless.

Another study, carried out by JECFA, the Joint FAO/WHO Expert Committee on Food Additives – the WHO is a member of it – showed in 1999, in experiments on rats over two years, that a daily intake at a concentration at a concentration of 2.5% (which corresponds to 970-1100 mg of stevioside per kilogram of body weight) is harmless.

The harmlessness of stevia was also determined by the ADI (= acceptable daily intake) value of the JECFA (including the WHO), and is therefore considered as harmless all over the world.

In decades of use of this plant, there has not been a single case of poisoning or health impairment.

The Guaraní Indians in South America have been using the stevia leaves for centuries – in considerable amounts every day. Today there is not a single case that would document that stevia somehow impaired their health. On the contrary, the Indians have practically no high blood pressure, are not overweight, have full hair, no heart diseases, and don't know diabetes.

What effect does stevia have on diabetes?

The plant has a positive influence on the blood sugar level. It improves the glucose tolerance. In the future, this might considerably reduce the increasing numbers of diabetes disease.

People who already suffer from diabetes also benefit from this plant. It can replace sugar.

Normal sugar is absorbed by the intestinal walls and gets into the blood almost in its entirety. In the case of stevia, absorption occurs through bacteria in the colon, which convert the chemical compound stevioside into steviole and sugar.

An average German consumes 150 grams of sugar a day. Replacing all this with stevia would result in an amount of 500 mg. This would result in only 250 mg of glucose. Only one-third of this gets into the blood circulation. Thus, the amount of glucose absorbed is less than 85 mg, compared to 150 grams of sugar.

It is notable that approximately three-fourths of the sugar consumed every day is "hidden" in foods: prepared meals, tomato ketchup, pickled cucumbers, meats and sausages, fruity yoghurt, etc.; sugar often has a conserving function in these cases.

An interesting study about nutrition in the case of diabetes

The university in Newcastle has published an interesting study. Since overweight is considered a major risk factor to get diabetes type 2, the volunteers, which suffered from recently acquired diabetes, were put on an 8-week diet with healthy foods, which among other things, included stevia.

The fat values got normalized with the diet. The insulin production increased. After 3 months, 7 of the 11 volunteers were healthy again.

If you sweeten your foods with stevia instead of sugar and put into practice a reduction of your calorie intake, the major risk factor of overweight is eliminated. In these cases, your body can activate the self-healing processes, and your diabetes will improve over time, up to a complete recovery.

These foods, combined with stevia, drastically reduce your blood sugar level

In total, over 100 active substances are known worldwide which can help reduce the blood sugar naturally. They only help type 2 diabetics, since insulin can still be formed. General mechanisms are stimulating insulin production, strengthening the effect (or both), and the substances achieve a delayed absorption of carbohydrates from the intestines into the blood, making the blood level increase slower. Below is a selection of foods with favorable effects on the blood sugar level.

Using the listed foods and consistently replacing sugar with stevia, you can keep diabetes type 2 under control.

Try to include more of these foods into your nutrition, and you'll get long-term results. There are numerous recipes which you can consume with stevia and with the foods listed here.

I like to refer people to the recipe collection of my esteemed colleague, Katharina Morell. Look in a good bookstore for her name, or under "recipes to lose weight", and you'll find diverse books with recipes which promote health. All recipes include stevia as sweetener.

Aloe Vera

Aloe Vera affects the insulin sensitivity and thus helps in reducing the blood sugar level.

Apples

The pectin contained in apples delays the absorption of sugar from foods in the blood. Pectin also protects the intestines and the blood vessels. Apples also contain a lot of vitamin C, flavones, carotene, vitamin B, potassium, calcium, phosphorus, iron and sodium. These substances are directly under the skin, therefore it is important to eat apples with their skin. It may be worthwhile to buy bio-apples, which you can eat unhesitatingly with their skin.

Avocado

Avocado does contain up to 30% fat, but ca. three-quarters of the fat consists of double-unsaturated fatty acids. Avocado contains lots of vitamins and minerals, especially vitamins A, C, and E, and the minerals potassium, calcium, copper, iron, and phosphorus. It also contains many B-vitamins, especial folic acid and pantothenic acid. It increases the insulin sensitivity and reduces insulin resistance.

Bananas

Bananas contain 10 different vitamins and 18 different minerals. When they are completely ripe, they contain a lot of fructose and glucose. If they are still slightly unripe, instead of sugar they have more starch, which is better for diabetics. Both the increase of blood sugar and of insulin gets reduced after eating bananas.

Bitter melon

This plant from India contains ingredients such as charantine and momordine as well as many vitamins and minerals. The ingredients charantine and momordine act similarly to insulin, reducing the blood sugar level. Momordine delays the absorption of carbohydrates in the intestines and helps to slow down the increase of the blood sugar level after eating.

Fenugreek

Fenugreek contains vitamins A, B1-B3 and C, as well as iron and phosphorus, saponine, mucilage and bitter substances. It helps reduce the blood sugar concentration, without increasing the insulin concentration.

Nettles

A tea from this plant stimulates the formation of insulin and delays the increase of blood sugar levels after a meal.

Grapefruit

In citrus fruits, but especially in grapefruit, a bitter substance was discovered – naringine. This bitter substance improves the insulin sensitivity and reduces blood fat values. Naringine has an effect similar to the commercial lipid (fat) reducers and medications that reduce blood sugar.

Prickly pear

Both the fruits and the leaf sprouts of this plant can be consumed; you can also get a powder on the market. The prickly pear makes the blood sugar level after a meal increase slower and improves the insulin effect. The plant thins the blood and should therefore be avoided by patients who are already taking blood-thinning medication. The cholesterol level is affected positively.

Cherries

Cherries contain many antioxidants and are rich in fiber. They also have only few calories and stimulate the body to produce insulin, thus reducing the risk to get diabetes.

Rattan vine

This plant comes from the south Indian forest. It increases the effect of insulin and reduces the increase of the blood sugar level after eating. Just 400 mg a day reduce the blood sugar level when on an empty stomach, and the long-term blood sugar value, measured over the HbA1C-value (a property of red blood cells).

Garlic

Raw garlic helps reduce the blood sugar level. Insulin production is stimulated; insulin sensibility is improved as well. Garlic also has antioxidant properties.

Flax seeds

Flax seeds are an important ingredient of a diabetes therapy. Flax seeds reduce the cholesterol level and reduce blood pressure. It doesn't contain many carbohydrates, but it does contain lots of minerals, omega-3 fatty acids and a significant amount of natural secondary vegetal ingredients.

Nuts

Nuts contain good fats and valuable proteins. They free long-lasting energy in the organism. Consuming a hand full of nuts every day can avoid insulin resistance. The risk of getting type 2 diabetes can be reduced by 20%. Especially appropriate are peanuts and walnuts, but also macadamia nuts are very valuable.

Sweet potatoes

Sweet potatoes not only reduce the blood sugar level, they are also valuable for health in general. Among other things, they contain beta-carotene and fibers. They increase insulin sensitivity and stabilize the blood sugar level.

Cinnamon

Cinnamon contains lots of magnesium and fiber, as well as the substance polyphenol, which has a similar effect in the body as insulin. Studies show that just a teaspoon daily of cinnamon reduces the blood sugar level up to 29%. The effect can persist up to 3 weeks. The cholesterol level is also affected favorably.

Lemons

Lemons are especially appropriate to regulate the blood sugar level. The fruit acid regulates the glycemic index; lemon also contains lots of vitamin C and rutin.

Onions

In onions, substances such as sulfur and flavonoids have an active effect in reducing the blood sugar level.

Green tea and cocoa

Green tea and cocoa (bitter chocolate) are also foods that reinforce the effect of insulin.

Known stevia products, available commercially as a sugar substitute

Industrially, stevia is advancing. Thus, the company Haribo offers stevi-licorice with 40% less calories. This confection is appropriate and even healthy for diabetics, since it is rich in fiber.

Pulmoll has changed its entire line of sugar-free sweets to stevia, and removed sweeteners known to be harmful, such as aspartame and the sweetener acesulfam K.

After several years of research, the dairy Andechser has released yoghurt with stevia on the market.

The drink manufacturer Coca-Cola has released calorie-reduced lemonades with stevia in the USA and in France; there are plans for Germany.

It is to be expected that stevia's importance for food will continue increasing. In the health area, many beneficial properties are already known, but the mechanisms are not completely clarified, and not all substances it contains have been discovered. Thus, in the future additional positive developments are to be expected.

Where, and in what form, is stevia available?

Stevia is available commercially as powder, tab, granules, tablets, dispersive powder, sugar-sticks, instant or liquid.

Just type the term "purchase stevia" in a search engine, and you'll find several websites where you can buy the miracle substance. Of course you can also buy "stevia" over Amazon, usually cheaper than in many other Web shops.

However, please pay attention to the instructions on the package about the dosage; every form has a different concentration; in the next chapter you'll find a conversion from sugar to stevia.

In Germany, Stevia products are verified in a nationally-certified German laboratory for purity of steviolglycosides, pesticide and heavy metal residua and microbes; thus, there is no risk in purchasing stevia.

Stevia powder has a green color. If you add stevia to foods or drinks, they will take on this green color. If you don't like this, you can use white extract powder or colorless stevia extract.

Sometimes you can get a bitter taste; in this case, the stevia dose is too high, and the sweet taste gets bitter.

There are stevia varieties on the market which have a taste similar to licorice. This is typical for the original plant. In the meantime, there are also stevia cultures that have a neutral taste.

Example of conversion from sugar to stevia

Since very form of stevia has a different concentration, you should always read through the instructions on the packing. The conversion refers to Stevia Sana products.

You can apply approximately the following conversions:

10 grams of sugar correspond to 1 measuring spoon (0.1 ml) of Stevia Sana liquid.

10 drops of Stevia Sana liquid converted to powder are 0.03 grams.

100 gram sugar correspond to 10 measuring spoons of Stevia Sana powder = 0.33 gram = 100 drops of Stevia Sana liquid.

Healthy stevia recipes which indulge the palate

Whether it is drinks, desserts, marmalades, fruit salad or sweet-sour foods, more and more stevia recipes make using the sweet plant simple and uncomplicated, so that your appetite for sweets must no longer go along with a guilty conscience.

If you like to experiment and consider recipes to be superfluous, it is recommended to be careful in the dosage, and preferably add extra sweetener later if so required.

Important: stevia is not appropriate for caramelizing; other than that, you can use stevia for cooking and baking just as sugar.

If you are affected by overweight or diabetes, I recommend the books by Katharina Morell, which you can find in good bookstores.

Try out the following recipes, to get a taste for it.

Egg pancakes

Mix 3 eggs with 50 ml soy milk and 5 teaspoons of stevia powder. Add a pinch of salt and beat with a whisk.

Put all this into a pan heated with some coconut oil and fry on medium heat.

When the pancake can be lifted easily, turn it around and finish frying it. You can put fresh applesauce on it, which you also sweeten slightly with stevia.

Vanilla cream

Mix 40 grams of food starch with a few tablespoons of milk (taken out of half a liter). Make the remaining milk cook with 50 drops of stevia.

Add a vanilla pod, cut in halves, to the milk, including the vanilla pulp. As soon as the milk is boiling, take the two half vanilla pods out again.

Add the mixed food starch to the milk; make it boil briefly.

Next put the cream into small bowls or glasses, let it cool and put it briefly into the refrigerator.

Before serving, the cream can be decorated with a fresh leaf of mint and a small fruit, depending on your tastes and the season.

Lemonade

Press the juice of 1-2 lemons and mix it with 10-14 leveled measuring spoons of Stevia Sana stevioside.

From a bottle of mineral water, pour out a small amount and slowly add the juice-stevia mix.

Attention: if you fill it in too quickly, the lemonade will bubble out of the bottle.

Banana ice cream

Mash 500 grams of completely ripe bananas and mix them with the juice of a lime.

Add 250 ml of low-fat milk, 150 ml of cream and half a knife point of stevia, briefly mix with a mixer and then place into an ice cream machine.

Lime-yoghurt cream

Wash 3 untreated limes. Rub off the peel of 2 limes and then put it aside. Then press out the limes.

Heat up the freshly pressed lime juice with 3 drops of stevia liquid. While doing this, soak 7 grams of leaf gelatin. Press out the gelatin and, while mixing it, make it dissolve in the lime-stevia mix.

Next stir in 250 grams of yoghurt and the rubbed-off peel of the 2 limes. Refrigerate this for ca. 30 minutes.

In the meantime, whip 250 grams of cream with 2 drops of stevia liquid until it is stiff, and also refrigerate it.

When the lemon-yoghurt mass is cooled down, mix in the cream.

Cut the third lime into slices. Fill out the lime cream in glasses, and adorn the cream with lime slices, a mint leaf and 2 fresh forest berries.

Choco-brownies

Separate 2 eggs and whip the white of the eggs. Break up 30 grams of couverture chocolate (light-bitter) into small pieces and make it melt with 55 grams of butter (for example, in the microwave oven, or in a water bath).

Mix 40 grams of cocoa powder with the butter-cocoa mix using a mixer, and mix in the 70 grams of almond powder, ½ teaspoon of baking powder, 1 bottle of vanilla flavor and 1 teaspoon of Stevia Chrystal Backsüße.

The mass will now get very solid! Carefully stir in the egg snow.

Fill in the mass into a 20x20 cm brownie form (or a similar casserole form) and smooth it out.

Bake it for ca. 20 minutes at 170 °C under-heat/over-heat.

Final comments

Just considering the economic damage caused by an increased number of diabetes cases, stevia can contribute significantly to improve people's health and to cause an economic relief for health insurance.

Numerous other diseases benefit from the plant's positive health benefits.

The delay in allowing the plant as a food additive in the EU is proof of how lobbyists of powerful groups (sugar and sweetener industries) are able to keep up their status – at the cost of people's health.

In the case of diabetes, nutrition is an important part of therapy. Unlike type 2 diabetics, type 1 diabetics are somewhat limited in their options to improve their situation through diet, due to the complete lack of insulin. For them, the intensified diabetes therapy has caused an improvement in their life quality.

Type 2 diabetics can considerably improve their life situation with nutrition, if they reduce their overweight, make use of general nutrition recommendations and use stevia as a sugar substitute.

For people who suffer from a previous stage of type 2 diabetes, chances are very good to live an entire life without insulin substitution, with some initiative and with only a few restrictions.

Even type 2 diabetics can get out of insulin substitution, if they consistently use stevia and foods that affect the blood sugar level.

I now wish you success for fighting against diabetes.

Sincerly Dr. Matt Roberts

www.ingramcontent.com/pod-product-compliance
Lightning Source LLC
Chambersburg PA
CBHW070937290526
45795CB00003B/1052